Table of Contents

What are Cannabis Edibles?

Cannabis edibles are food or beverages that have been infused with cannabis compounds, primarily tetrahydrocannabinol (THC) or cannabidiol (CBD). Unlike smoking or vaping cannabis, edibles offer an alternative method of consuming cannabis that does not involve inhalation. Edibles can come in various forms, including baked goods, candies, chocolates, beverages, and more. They offer a discreet and convenient way to experience the effects of cannabis.

Cannabis edibles are typically created by infusing cannabis extracts or oils into the cooking or baking process. The cannabinoids present in the cannabis plant, such as THC or CBD, bind to the fat or oil in the recipe, allowing for their absorption by the body upon ingestion. The effects of cannabis edibles can be different from those of smoking or vaping, as the cannabinoids are metabolized by the liver and released into the bloodstream over a more extended period.

1.2 Benefits of Cannabis Edibles

Cannabis edibles offer several advantages over other forms of cannabis consumption:

a) Longer-lasting effects: When cannabis is ingested, the effects tend to last longer compared to smoking or vaping. The cannabinoids are processed by the liver and released gradually into the bloodstream, resulting in a prolonged and more balanced experience.

b) Discreet consumption: Edibles provide a discreet way to consume cannabis without the need for smoking or carrying paraphernalia. They resemble regular food items, making them inconspicuous and suitable for those who prefer a more private experience.

c) Precise dosing: Edibles allow for precise dosing, as the THC or CBD content is measured and evenly distributed across the entire batch. This makes it easier to control the amount of cannabis consumed, ensuring a consistent and predictable experience.

d) Variety of options: Cannabis edibles offer a wide range of options in terms of flavors, textures, and types of food or beverages. Whether you prefer sweet treats, savory snacks, or refreshing drinks, there is a vast selection of edibles available to cater to different tastes and preferences.

1.3 Legal Considerations

It is essential to understand the legal considerations surrounding cannabis edibles, as laws and regulations vary from one jurisdiction to another. While the legalization of cannabis for recreational or medicinal use has expanded in many places, it is crucial to familiarize yourself with the specific laws in your region.

In some areas, cannabis edibles may be fully legal and readily available for purchase from licensed dispensaries. However, there may be restrictions on the THC content per serving or packaging requirements to ensure proper labeling and child-resistant packaging.

In other regions, the use and distribution of cannabis edibles may be more restricted. Some jurisdictions may only allow the use of CBD-infused edibles or limit the purchase and consumption of THC-infused edibles to medical cannabis patients. It is essential to research and comply with the regulations in your area to avoid any legal consequences.

Additionally, it is vital to keep cannabis edibles out of reach of children and pets, as they can mistake them for regular food items. Proper storage, clear labeling, and responsible consumption are crucial to ensuring the safety of everyone in your household.

Always consult local laws and regulations and adhere to them when using or creating cannabis edibles. It is your responsibility to stay informed and make informed decisions regarding the use and legality of cannabis in your jurisdiction.

By understanding what cannabis edibles are, appreciating their benefits, and being aware of legal considerations, you are better equipped to explore this exciting and evolving world. In the following sections, we will dive deeper into the science of cannabis, dosage and safety guidelines, and the art of cooking with cannabis to enhance your knowledge and enjoyment of cannabis edibles.

A BEGINNERS GUIDE TO CANNABIS EDIBLES

Cannabis edibles can be a wonderful, discreet, delicious way to consume cannabis, but they can also pose potential safety concerns if not done responsibly.

Unlike traditional smoking or vaporizing, edibles have a more potent and powerful intoxicating effect for many people.

Additionally, cannabis edibles have a delayed onset of 90-minutes to several hours, making it extremely difficult to predict the onset time, dose-response, and duration of the experience.

Of course, cannabis edibles are meant to be enjoyed and can be an excellent addition to and healthy lifestyle with some basic education.

By following these few safe edible recommendations below, you can ensure you are prepared to have an experience that is safe, positive, and rewarding.

THE IMPORTANCE OF DECARBOXYLATION

Before getting started, it is important to note that all raw or dried cannabis must undergo a process called decarboxylation to be able to enjoy the active forms of CBD or THC.

Raw and dried cannabis flower contains what is known as tetrahydrocannabinolic acid (THCA) and cannabidiolic acid (CBDA).

These cannabinoids are found in the raw cannabis plant material and contain their own powerful health benefits.

However, these cannabinoids are not intoxicating in their natural state. Decarboxylation is a process that converts THCa → Δ9-THC and CBDa → CBD.

Using heat and/or solvents is the most common way to decarboxylate the cannabis flower before enjoying it.

Mastering the process of cannabis decarboxylation is an important skill to have for anyone who wants to infuse their own cannabis recipes home.

Decarboxylation Summary: When making cannabis edibles, it is important to decarboxylate your cannabis material before consuming it in order to reap the full benefits of activated CBD or THC.

UNDERSTANDING EDIBLES DELAYED ONSET

It can be difficult, potentially dangerous, and sometimes time-consuming for you to find your ideal cannabis edible dosage.

One reason being the delayed onset time of cannabis consumption to produce the desired effect.

It is even more difficult to determine how the consumed product will affect you and how long the effects will last.

The experience varies widely from person to person thanks to our own unique endocannabinoid system (ECS).

It can be difficult to determine your ideal dosage when orally consuming cannabis because the onset of the desired effect is significantly delayed compared to sublingual, topical, or inhalation administration routes.

Orally ingested cannabis is slower to take effect, with the typical onset time ranging anywhere from 30 minutes to 2 hours, or even longer, depending on the individual.

While the effects of consumed cannabis are delayed, they tend to manifest stronger and last longer with a peak onset of noticeable effects setting between 1 to 3 hours post-consumption.

The effects of cannabis edibles can last anywhere from 6 to 8 hours or more and vary gratefully from person to person.

It is important to remember that cannabinoids like CBD and THC are eaten have anywhere from a 6-10% bioavailability rate.

Individual physiological factors, such as absorption rates, rates of metabolism and excretion, and body weight, can affect the bioavailability of cannabinoids that also vary from person to person.

Edibles Delayed Onset Summary: Consuming cannabis edibles have a much longer delayed onset time than traditionally inhaling cannabis. The onset time of intoxicating effects can be anywhere from 30 minutes to 2 hours, peak experience from 1 to 3 hours, and duration lasting 6 to 8 hours or more post-consumption.

EDIBLES CAN BE MORE POTENT

Orally consuming cannabis will indeed provide stronger, more potent, or intoxicating effects in some individuals.

There are anecdotal reports of people experiencing hallucinogenic effects in some situations where too much THC has been orally consumed.

The edible consumption method is different from inhaling or topical administration.

Once the cannabis is eaten and digested, the THC is absorbed into the bloodstream and travels to the liver, where it undergoes the hepatic first-pass metabolism.

During this process, enzymes hydroxylate Δ9-THC to form 11-hydroxytetrahydrocannabinol (11-OH-THC), a potent psychoactive metabolite that readily crosses the blood-brain barrier.

This potent intoxicating metabolite causes potentially unwanted (or wanted) side effects for many unknowing cannabis consumers.

It is important to note that a portion of the population report feeling no effect from cannabis edibles at all.

This may be because they lack the enzyme (or enough of the enzymes) needed to convert Δ9-THC → 11-OH-THC.

Edibles Can Be More Potent Summary: When cannabis is eaten, it goes through the digestive system. As it goes through the liver, Δ9-THC is hydroxylated to 11-OH-THC, a potent psychoactive metabolite that readily crosses the blood-brain barrier. It is this intoxicating metabolite that causes more potent, increased intoxicating effects with cannabis edibles.

DETERMINING FINAL PRODUCT POTENCY

For many cannabis consumers, the most difficult piece of the oral cannabis consumption puzzle is accurately assessing their final product's potency to understand their final dosages.

It is nearly impossible to determine the exact concentration of final cannabinoids like CBD and THC without lab testing when making an at-home recipe, like the staple cannabis coconut oil or cannabis butter.

This is a disadvantage for you because it is nearly impossible to accurately assess and track how much of each cannabinoid you will be orally consuming.

This uncertainty opens up the risk of you either underdosing or overdosing, which will ultimately prevent you from experiencing your edibles' desired health benefits.

It can help if you know the strain and cannabinoid concentrations of your cannabis product before cooking.

For example, if the flower was purchased at a dispensary, it may say 22% THC, 4% CBD.

If you have this information, a few calculations may help you to guestimate your final product potency.

Determining Final Product Potency Summary: Without knowing the concentration of CBD or THC in your starting material, and without lab testing, it is nearly impossible to estimate the final potency of your homemade cannabis edibles.

SAFETY CONSIDERATIONS FOR CONSUMING THC EDIBLES

I always encourage my Cannabis Compass students to prepare their own medicinal oils, butter, edibles, or capsules at home for many reasons, including the cost savings and flexibility with personal preferences.

Consuming CBD oil in food does not pose much of a risk, and making homemade CBD gummies is unlikely to produce any intoxicating effects.

It is when you are working with THC dominant strains that you begin to run the risk of accidentally experiencing an intoxicating or even a hallucinogenic effect if the enzymes in your liver hydroxylate Δ9-THC to form 11-OH-THC, the potent intoxicating metabolite mentioned above.

Consuming too much THC can pose a safety risk, mainly for unsuspecting individuals.

The most common unwanted side effects that may pose a safety risk to some individuals include:

- Disorientation or dizziness

- Short-term memory issues

- Slow reaction time

- Drowsiness

- Anxiety

- Heart-palpitations

- Tachycardia (rapid heartbeat)

- Increased appetite with dry mouth[1]

THC Safety Considerations Summary: Unknowingly consuming too much THC, especially in the form of cannabis edibles, may result in disorientation, dizziness, drowsiness, anxiety, and tachycardia.

EDIBLES ARE BOTH AN EXPERIMENT & COMMITMENT

Consuming cannabis edibles is truly a self-experiment that requires both curiosity and patience.

It will likely take several tries for you to find a dosage with an identifiable onset and duration time that you can rely on.

For this reason, I always recommend to my Cannabis Compass Course students that they consume cannabis edibles in the safety of their own home when they have a significant amount of time, at least 24 hours, to stay put and comfortably enjoy the experience.

Experimenting with dosages and duration times requires a time commitment from yourself.

With the notoriously delayed onset and duration time of edibles, you should plan on devoting at least 6-12 hours to your experience.

During this time, plan to be safe in your home with no need to travel anywhere, no driving a car, and no operating heavy machinery.

Edibles Are a Commitment Summary: The delayed onset time and unknown intoxicating response meaning that it may take a few tries for you to find your perfect dose or edible recipe. Consuming cannabis edibles is both a self-experiment and a time commitment.

DOSING RECOMMENDATIONS FOR BEGINNERS

With cannabis, there is no such thing as standard dosing recommendations, as cannabis affects everyone differently.

Everyone's body metabolizes cannabis differently.

You and your identical twin could consume the same teaspoon of cannabis tincture and have drastically different experiences.

It is important to start with one low dose first and to monitor your body's reaction.

I repeat, begin with one very low dose to start with (>5mg THC if you know the final potency).

Remember, cannabis edibles can have a delayed onset time of 30-minutes to 2 hours or more, so don't take a second dose after just one hour, or you risk the chance of consuming more than you can comfortably handle.

If you do not feel any response after four hours, then gradually titrate up the dose and try again.

Remember to record the amount you took before you take it, so you can go back and compare dosages if needed.

Dosage Recommendations Summary: There is no standard dosage recommendation for cannabis edibles. Start LOW and go SLOW. Try a small amount first and gradually titrate up as needed. Your patience will be rewarded with a safe, enjoyable experience.

IMPORTANT: TAKE NOTES AFTER CONSUMING!

If you are new to cannabis edibles and are using cannabis to improve your health, it is essential to take notes on each cannabis edible experience to learn from each experience.

This will help you to repeat the good experiences and avoid bad experiences and allow you to track your dosages and progress over time.

HOW TO MAKE CANNABUTTER

Cannabis butter, also called cannabutter, is likely the most tried and true cannabis-infused recipe known to the culinary cannabis world.

I've covered cannabis coconut oil, cannabis olive oil, and cannabis tinctures here on the blog.

Still, after seeing hundreds of searches on my site for cannabutter, I knew it was time to deliver.

Cannabis butter, or cannabutter, is one of the essential cannabis recipes for anyone looking to make their edibles at home because it is versatile and easy to make.

Once you have your cannabis butter made, you can use it in just about any recipe you can dream of that traditionally calls for butter.

From sweet to savory recipes, like classic brownies and cannabis chocolate chip cookies, there is a use for cannabis butter in just about every recipe you can imagine.

It is easy to make your cannabis butter at home, and it can save you a lot of money compared to pricey automatic butter makers, although they can be super convenient for some users.

IF YOU ARE NEW TO CANNABIS EDIBLES

If you are brand new to cannabis edibles, I want to make sure you check out my Beginners Guide to Cannabis Edibles first.

Homemade edibles can be difficult to dose, and often more potent than any other type of cannabis consumption.

Friends don't let friends go into edibles unprepared, so let me help you!

Grab my cannabis edibles guide here.

If you are brand new to cannabis in general and are looking for foundational knowledge about your endocannabinoid system, I offer a more in-depth educational session inside my Cannabis Compass Online Course.

If you've never cooked with cannabis before, I recommend experimenting with CBD hemp flower first, as it is usually easier to access and cheaper to buy.

Experimenting with a more affordable CBD hemp flower also means less heartache if there ever happens to be a mistake made along the way.

BEFORE YOU GET STARTED

Just keep in mind that there is no 'right way' to cook with cannabis.

While some guidelines you should generally stick with, many chefs have different techniques when cooking with cannabis.

It is OK for you to develop your preferred method, too, as long as you end up with the outcome you desire.

General Guidelines:

1. Choose your decarboxylation (or decarb) process

2. Don't use margarine or other types of 'fake' butter

3. Be careful not to overheat the butter while cooking

Please join my Well With Cannabis Facebook Community if you have any questions about cooking with cannabis, making cannabis butter, how to make this recipe specifically, or anything else you can think of!

CHOOSE YOUR DECARB PROCESS

Raw cannabis flower does not naturally contain high amounts of THC or CBD, but it does contain high amounts of cannabinoid acids THCA and CBDA, part of the full-spectrum of cannabinoids.

To experience the intoxicating 'high' effect of cannabis, you want to convert that CBDA and THCA into CBD and THC, respectively, with a process called decarboxylation.

Decarboxylation can occur with heat and/or solvents.

There are two primary ways to decarboxylate when making cannabutter.

The first method involves decarboxylating the cannabis in the oven before infusing with the butter.

The second method involves allowing the cannabis butter to cook for twice as long using fat for the solvent, allowing decarboxylation to occur over time.

OPTION 1: DECARB IN THE OVEN

This option is preferred because it cuts your cooking time in half.

Before infusing the cannabis and the butter together, you will first bake the dried cannabis flowers in the oven at 240° F for 40 minutes.

After baking, you will then combine the cooked flower with the butter and allow them to infuse together for 4 hours in a crockpot, slow cooker, or on the stovetop.

OPTION 2: DECARB WHILE COOKING

Some prefer this option because it eliminates the need to decarboxylate the flower in the oven ahead of time.

It's true, you can skip the step of decarboxylating in the oven, but it's important to note that you will need to cook the cannabis butter for an extended period of time to achieve full decarboxylation.

This option will also produce a more 'green' tasting product, as the longer cooking times will release more chlorophyll into the infusion.

FREQUENTLY ASKED QUESTIONS: HOW TO MAKE CANNABUTTER

Below I will break down some of the most frequently asked questions I get about how to make the best cannabutter recipe and hopefully share some tips along the way to help you make the best cannabutter possible.

WHY BUTTER?

There are both culinary and scientific reasons why butter is an excellent choice for making homemade edibles.

From a culinary perspective, butter is extremely versatile and can be used in so many recipes, ranging from sweet to savory dishes.

From a scientific perspective, cannabinoids are lipophilic, meaning that they dissolve in and bind to fat.

When cannabinoids are extracted with fat, they are more easily absorbed and thus more bioavailable in our bodies (1).

Most butter purchased from the grocery store is on average 80-82% milk fat, 16–17% water, and 1–2% milk solids, which are mostly protein and sometimes referred to as curd (2).

During the cooking process, we will evaporate the water and remove the milk solids, leaving a pure, infused butter.

WHAT TYPE OF BUTTER SHOULD I USE?

I recommend to use unsalted butter when making your cannabutter because it is less impurity in the butter itself.

While both salted or unsalted butter will work, many Chefs prefer infusing unsalted butter in general for cooking.

As a general rule of thumb, the higher quality of the butter you use to start, the higher quality your final product will be.

Kerrygold is a commonly recommended brand because the butter comes from the milk of grass-fed cows free of growth hormones.

Additionally, Kerrygold unsalted butter has a higher butterfat content, meaning more opportunity for cannabinoid infusion and fewer impurities to remove.

SHOULD I USE CLARIFIED BUTTER?

It is controversial among the culinary cannabis community on whether or not you should clarify your butter before starting the infusion process.

Some people say they never clarify first and make fabulous butter every time, while others say they would never make cannabutter without clarifying the butter first.

You can do it either way. You don't have to or need to clarify your butter. It's a preference most have, not a necessity.

For this recipe, we do not clarify the butter ahead of time, but simply separate the final infused butter from the leftover water and milk solids left behind from the cooking process at the end.

If you want to clarify your butter ahead of time, you would simply gently boil the butter in a saucepan over the stove and skim all the foam, or milk solids, from the top.

This process will also evaporate much of the water naturally present in butter.

Remember, if you clarify your butter, you will be losing approximately 15-20% of your total weight and volume.

If you already have clarified butter, follow this cannabis coconut oil recipe and simply swap the cannabis coconut oil for your clarified butter.

WHAT IS THE WHITE STUFF?

If you do not clarify your butter first, you will notice white particles on your cooked butter.

The white stuff is nothing to be alarmed about; the white particles are simply the milk solids and salt if you used salted butter.

These solids will be removed when we strain and discard the excess water.

WHAT ABOUT GHEE?

Ghee is butter that has already been clarified or has had the milk solids removed. This pre-done step eliminates the need for you to clarify your butter.

In this clarified state, ghee is essentially an oil and can be cooked like a traditional cannabis oil infusion.

Use this cannabis coconut oil recipe and simply swap the cannabis coconut oil for your ghee to make simple cannabis-infused ghee.

WHY DID I END UP WITH LESS BUTTER THAN I STARTED WITH?

As mentioned above, you will lose weight and volume in the cooking process and end up with less butter than you started with.

The loss occurs because you will be removing the milk solids and evaporating off the excess water.

You should expect to experience a volume loss of 15-25%.

Volume loss is essential to keep in mind, especially if you try to make a small batch to use in a particular recipe.

For example, one stick of butter that has been infused is no longer still one stick of butter typically called for in a recipe.

DO I NEED A THERMOMETER?

Yes, we recommend using an instant digital read thermometer for monitoring your temperature accurately.

You risk denaturing or destroying the essential cannabinoids and terpenes at temperatures that are too high.

HOW LONG TO COOK CANNABUTTER IN THE CROCKPOT?

You will cook your cannabutter in the crockpot for 4-hours with pre-decarbed cannabis and 8-hours with non-decarbed cannabis.

CAN I COOK CANNABUTTER IN A PAN OF BOILING WATER?

Yes, you can.

For this recipe, we are using a crockpot because it is easier to maintain a constant temperature and 'set-it-and-forget-it', but the truth is you don't need any special equipment like a crockpot at all.

To cook your cannabutter without a crockpot, place the decarboxylated cannabis flowers, unsalted butter, and 2 cups of water in a medium-sized saucepan.

Bring to a boil and allow to cook on the stovetop for 4 hours. Once the cooking process is over, simply allow the entire pan to cool.

The finished butter will harden and solidify, or float, on top, while the unwanted water will remain on the bottom.

Simply pour off the water and discard it, and you will be left with your final product.

DO I NEED TO ADD WATER?

You do not need to add water to the mason jars if you are cooking in a crockpot, but you will be using a water bath.

When cooking in a crockpot, a water bath helps to maintain a constant temperature.

You will need to add water to the pot if you are cooking your butter on the stovetop.

When cooking on a stovetop, the temperature can fluctuate quite a bit.

The water helps to regulate the temperature of the butter, preventing it from getting too hot and ultimately burning your butter and denaturing your cannabinoids.

*Note: If you add water to your cannabutter infusion, do NOT add lecithin as well.

This will bind the water and butter together, resulting in a soupy mess.

DO I NEED TO USE A MASON JAR?

We used a mason jar in the crockpot here for ease and convenience, but you don't need to.

If you are using the stovetop method above, you can simply combine everything in the saucepan without putting anything in a mason jar.

If you are cooking in a mason jar, note that there can be an occasional mishap that results in a broken or cracked jar – it happens to the best of us without rhyme or reason.

Some tips to help prevent this:

1. Use mason jars specifically meant for canning or cooking. Do not use leftover glass jars from other products

2. Make sure you use new mason jars with a brand new lid so you know the

seal is good and the contents inside will stay dry

We used two of these 16 ounce wide-mouth Ball mason jars in this recipe, and they fit perfectly inside this 7-quart crockpot we use.

WHAT IF MY MASON JAR FLOATS?

Sometimes the mason jar will float when placed in the water bath.

Floating jars are no need for concern. Simply add something heat and water safe over the top of the jar to weigh it down; a clean rock works well.

CAN I SOUS VIDE CANNABIS BUTTER?

Yes you can make sous vide cannabutter.

If you have an immersion circulator, you will follow the same process and set your water bath to a temperature of 185° F and cook for the same amount of time, approximately 4 hours with a pre-decarbed flower or 8 hours with non-decarbed flower.

CAN I JUST USE A CANNABUTTER MAKER?

Yes, if you don't want to make your cannabutter in a crockpot or stovetop, you can try a cannabutter maker, also known as a cannabutter machine.

Popular cannabutter machines on the market today include the Magic Butter Machine and the Levo Infusion Machine.

WHAT TYPE OF WEED SHOULD I USE?

Well, the truth is, anything you can get your hands on will work.

For some people, that means trim and shake, and for others, it means high-quality bud purchased at a legal dispensary.

All parts of the cannabis plant, aside from the stems and seeds, contain some cannabinoids that can be infused into butter.

Some parts of the plant, like the buds, contain more cannabinoids than other parts, like the trim leaves.

Here are the most popular options to work with. Keep in mind that how much you use will also impact your final potency:

HIGH-QUALITY CANNABIS FLOWER

Using high-quality dried cannabis flower buds will make a stronger, more potent butter because the flower bud contains a high concentration of cannabinoids.

CANNABUTTER MADE WITH TRIM LEAVES AND SHAKE

Using up all parts of the cannabis plant is great for sustainability. Trim, leaves, and shake all contain varying amounts of cannabinoids.

Because leaves do not contain nearly as many cannabinoids as flower buds, you may want to consider using more trim, leaves, and shake than you would flower.

HOW TO MAKE KIEF BUTTER

Kief is the fine, powdery substance that accumulates at the bottom of a grinder contains the resinous glands that have the most cannabinoids from the trichomes.

Because kief is so much more potent, you may be able to use less of it in this recipe, depending on the effect you're looking for. Just remember that you still need to decarb kief just as you would traditional flower.

HOW DO I MAKE MY CANNABUTTER STRONGER?

The potency of your final cannabis butter is directly related to the potency of the starting cannabis flower you started with, your decarb process, and your cooking process.

With the decarbing and cooking process spelled out here, the one variable you have the most control over is your starting material.

Remember, the better the bud, the better the butter. You can also try an online cannabutter ratio calculator if you're feeling stuck.

TO MAKE A MORE POTENT CANNABIS BUTTER:

1. Choose a higher-quality flower that contains more % THC

2. Add kief, or cannabis concentrates like distillate or FECO

3. Use more flowers (an increase from 1 ounce to 2 ounces or more)

4. Use less butter (decrease from 1 pound to 1/2 pound)

HOW DO I KNOW HOW POTENT MY FINAL BATCH IS?

Spoiler alert – it is challenging to estimate the potency of homemade edibles if you do not know the % concentrations of THCA, THC, or CBDA, CBD in your starting flower without lab testing.

If you know the % concentration of your starting flower (easier if you purchased from a dispensary or know the actual strain), you can use an online calculator to guestimate your final product potency.

Again, the potency will depend on the strength of the flower you start with.

If you have no clue the starting potency of your material, it's best to start with a low dose when consuming your first batch, to be able to get a better understanding of how strong the product is and how it makes you feel.

DOES THE FINAL GREEN COLOR OF THE BUTTER MATTER?

No, color doesn't have any correlation with potency.

A very green butter is simply a cannabis butter with a lot of chlorophyll, the green pigment that has also been extracted from the plant.

You will likely have more chlorophyll and green color if you are making the butter with trim, and the fresher the bud, the greener it will also be.

WHAT SHOULD I USE TO STRAIN?

We always recommend using something that is food-grade safe to strain your cannabis butter.

We use a large paper oil filter and recommend a fine China cap strainer or clean, unbleached cheesecloth.

We do not recommend using anything that is not food-safe, like pantyhose.

WHAT CAN I DO WITH THE PULP?

Many people simply discard their cooked plant matter after straining their butter or oil.

Still, we've heard many success stories of people who have successfully used the pulp in another recipe with various intoxicating effects.

We believe in whole plant nutrition and sustainability, waste reduction, and repurposing where able.

We've experimented with cooking with the leftover cannabis pulp and have discovered that it can make a delightful addition to so many of your favorite dishes!

Here we have put together a round-up of all of the delicious ways we have successfully incorporated leftover plant matter from making cannabutter in this post featuring 15 Ways To Use Leftover Cannabis Pulp.

IN-DEPTH STEP-BY-STEP INSTRUCTIONS

The instructions above are concise and perfect for printing, but I have many students who like step-by-step instructions with pictures.

Here is a more in-depth, detailed guide of the entire process for those who need a bit more information than I provided above.

Step #1: Lay a clean tea towel down on the bottom of a large crockpot. This will create a buffer between your mason jars and the crockpot, potentially preventing any jar moving or cracking during cooking.

Step #2: Fill your crockpot with enough warm water to cover the mason jars you plan on using to create a water bath. Be careful not to overflow.

Step #3: Place a digital thermometer in the water and set the crockpot to high heat. When a temperature of around 185°F is reached, turn the heat to low.

Step #4: While the water bath is heating, measure, and decarb your cannabis flower by baking it in an oven set to 240° F for 40 minutes